Sick of Being Fat

Catherine Grace Cleveland

Nothing written in this book is intended as medical advice or as a substitute for competent medical care. Do not make changes in your diet or exercise plan without first consulting your physician or health care provider especially if you are already being treated for current medical issues.

Copyright © 2012 by Catherine Grace Cleveland

All rights reserved. No part of this book my be used or reproduced, copied, stored or transmitted electronically in any manner whatsoever without prior written permission from the publisher.

ISBN-13: 978-1468122718
ISBN-10: 1468122711

www.sickofbeingfat.info

To lose weight, you must be willing to make changes that you are not presently willing to make. This book encourages you to find your strength and power, to get what you deserve; a fit and healthy mind and body.

I am proud of myself for having the strength and courage to go against our society's norm of the disease-promoting American diet and embrace a healthy lifestyle. I am grateful to all my friends and colleagues who believe in me and support me, especially my love John P. Mann.

Contents

Introduction	11
Why 100% Plant Powered?	17
Why Diets Don't Work	21
How to Apply Plant Power	23
Foods to Eat	27
Your Primary Food Sources	31
Eat Enough to Meet Your Caloric Intake Needs	32
Beverages	32
Eat These Rarely or Preferably Never	33
Supplements	34
Read Food Labels	36
Food Elimination Chart	39
Explanation of the Food Elimination Chart	41
Meat, Fish, and Eggs	42
Dairy	43
Fast Food, Fried Food, and Pizza	45
Candy, Cookies, and Unhealthy Desserts	46
Soda, Energy Drinks, Fruit Juice, and Juice Drinks	46
Alcohol	47
Sugar	48
Caffeine	50

Oil and Fat	50
Sodium	51
Health Foods	51

Problems That You Can Run Into When
You Are Trying to Lose Weight 53
- Belief System — 53
- Addiction — 54
- Withdrawal — 56
- Exercise — 57
- Cravings — 58
- Stress — 59
- The Scale — 60
- The Dreaded Plateau — 61
- Clothing Expense — 62
- Doctors and Their Prescription Pads — 63
- Ridicule — 65
- Second-guessing Yourself — 69
- Excuses — 68
- Relapse — 70
- Hormones — 71
- Balance — 72

Cooking Advice 79
- Start a Garden — 80
- Get Your Kids Involved in Cooking — 81
- Eating Out — 82
- Meal Timing — 83
- Cooking Equipment — 85
- Foods to Have Available — 86

Power Food Recipes ... 91
   Lunch and Dinner Recipes ... 91
   Breakfast Recipes ... 107
   Sides ... 108
   Sweets and Snacks ... 114

Exercise Advice ... 119

The Importance of Nutritional Counseling ... 125

Summary ... 127

List of Notable Vegans ... 129

Resources ... 135

Introduction

In order to lose weight, you must start with an unwavering commitment to do what it takes to be successful. How much are you really willing to change to get what you want? True success in losing weight comes from making permanent changes to your lifestyle and in your environment.

I have years of experience in dieting defeat, as most of us who are overweight do. I understand the struggle of people who are overweight, especially the overindulging, worthlessness, and giving up. I have struggled with being overweight all my life. I was the fat kid back in the days when there were only one or two fat kids in the whole school. Now more than 35% of children are overweight and usually many of their family members are too. This is an epidemic that is destroying our health, financial well being, and quality of life.

Today, I have successfully lost all of my excess weight, I am healthy, I am not starving myself, I feel good, and I enjoy life more than ever. From my weight-loss journey and nutritional education, I have learned how our bodies and emotions respond to what we eat. One of the most important things that made me successful in losing weight and keeping it off was my own strong inner voice telling me that life can be enjoyed so much more by being fit and healthy.

My weight-loss battle started in my late teens. This was about the time that the relentless teasing I experienced started to affect my self-esteem. As most people who want to lose weight would do, I started seeking and listening to any weight-loss advice I could find. I would listen to stories of how people would lose their weight and the next thing you know, with the best intentions, I would open up my wallet and test the gimmick for myself. When I reached my thirties, fad diets were all the rage. The Atkins Diet! I lost ten pounds and I thought I was going to starve to death, not to mention it made me lightheaded and completely brain-fried from the lack of carbs. One of my favorites though, was the low-fat diet: just eat all the processed sugar you want. As I recall, I devoured boxes of SnackWell's and gained ten pounds. Take a look at how all those fad diets and fad diet pills are working today. More than 65% of Americans are overweight and obese and the numbers are increasing. Conclusion: Diets don't work, but you probably already knew that.

Entering my forties was a particularly tough time for me. My husband had been showing signs of becoming ill, mainly fatigue and short-term memory loss. We spent years and hundreds of thousands of dollars on doctor bills, hospital bills, and lost wages trying to figure out what was causing his memory loss, headaches, and insomnia. My husband was a fifth-generation dairy farmer, which exposed him to all sorts of chemicals. He also lived on ice cream, red meat, processed junk food, and an excessive amount of diet cola. After two years of brain scans, his doctors finally detected his brain tumor, but not until four weeks prior to his death. As a result of his chosen lifestyle, I believe he prematurely and unnecessarily died, but who knew?

For a long time after my husband's death, I was angry. Angry at myself for not being able to get him better, angry at my husband for not trying hard enough to live, and angry at all the healthcare providers (including today's corporate-owned TV doctors) who don't come clean about what is really causing reversible illnesses such as heart disease, diabetes, and cancer. Nevertheless, my life needed to go on and I didn't want to waste it being angry at the things I can't control. My husband's death was a big wake-up call for me and a big, hard kick in the pants to pay attention to the damage I was doing to myself through my bad eating habits and my chosen unhealthy lifestyle.

    I had an opportunity to start my life over, and I knew in my soul that I was determined to live the best life for me that I possibly could. I started with educating myself about nutrition and its effects, both good and bad. I began by taking nutrition and wellness courses and by listening to information in the media about certain foods that could be bad for you. If you haven't noticed, there is a constant media battle about what is healthy (good healthcare versus large food corporations) and what is not. No wonder people are so confused and misinformed. Studying about nutrition and its effects has created several opportunities for me, greatly improved my health, and helped me through my divesting mourning period. One of the most important lessons that I have learned from this is that nutrition really does affect all aspects of our lives.

    By eating strictly plant-based foods, I am feeling fantastic and I am 45 pounds lighter. I am 5'8" and weigh 130 pounds, and I am not obsessed with my weight anymore. I eat until I am full, and the weight does not come back on. I am 100% plant powered, meaning what I eat is what nature grows. I do not eat food that is processed, has added fat, is chemically altered, or has parents. I love what I eat and I feel great.

As you read this book, you will discover that it is not about being on a "diet." This is part of a nutritional education plan to help you get healthy, lose weight, and eliminate your addictions that keep sabotaging your success. There is no weighing, measuring, or counting points. This plan is easy to understand, but if you are not educated about nutrition and the effects that it has on your health, you might find it rather shocking, at least until you try it. Thriving on whole, plant-based food will eventually have you feeling and looking better, and you will stop being tired and sick all the time. Everyone will want to know how you did it, but when you tell them, they most likely won't be willing to jump on board.

Why 100% Plant Powered?

Being 100% plant powered or whole, plant-based is eating a diet that is healthy and the way nature intends it to be. Our bodies and brains are designed to grow, develop, and function on nutrients provided by nature. In the United States, our "American" diet consists of calorie-dense, processed, and chemically enhanced foods and food-like substances.

We have an obesity and chronic disease epidemic in this country that is so bad that young people believe that it is normal to have chronically ill and overweight family members, because most of the people that they know are. It is the "norm," but it is not normal. Simply put, bad nutrition equals bad health, and good nutrition equals good health.

About 80% of the major diseases in this country can be prevented by whole, plant-based diets and "healthy living" lifestyles. Whole, plant-based living can reverse diabetes and heart disease, and greatly help to reverse some cancers and many other chronic diseases. It will enable you to lose weight and keep it off. Eating whole, plant-based foods will make you feel better than you do now and will allow you to stop going on and off diets, binge eating and starving yourself.

If you have too much fat on your body, you are susceptible to developing a chronic disease if you don't already have one. As a result of being overweight and having chronic diseases, you will eventually end up in a hospital. You will most likely go under the knife and have other horrible and painful treatments, because you didn't learn, apply, or understand the importance that nutrition plays in your life.

Here is a list of things that can be prevented, cured, or greatly improved upon by adopting a whole, plant-based diet:

- Your weight
- Your blood pressure
- Heart disease, stroke, and diabetes
- Cancers
- Mood disorders, anxiety, anger, and depression
- Your sex life and erectile dysfunction
- ADD and ADHD
- Dementia and Alzheimer's disease
- Your quality of life
- Stress

- Constipation
- PMS
- Menopause
- Cold sores
- Your cost of living, such as saving money on junk food, supplements, doctors, hospitals, and unnecessary prescriptions
- Daytime fatigue
- Tooth decay
- Dermatitis (helps clear up acne).

Some of the benefits of a whole, plant-based diet include the following:
- You can reduce your carbon footprint.
- You will look and feel younger.
- You will have constant energy and feel empowered.
- You can live simpler and improve your outlook on life.
- You can age more slowly and be more functional.
- It could save your life.

Have you heard of plaque in your arteries? Before I started eating whole, plant-based foods, I was living fat on the American diet. I remember what it was like trying to do the dishes. You know the baked-on, cheesy, greasy fat, the stuff that relentlessly sticks to your dishes? That's the same garbage that you eat, and it builds plaque in your arteries. It can kill you. Plant-based cleanup is a breeze. You will notice the difference right away and so will your hardening arteries.

For more inspiration to go plant based check out Vegsource (www.vegsource.com) and Rip Esselstyn's interview on (http://www.youtube.com/watch?v=y_DEv2w8YQE).

Why Diets Don't Work

Diets are temporary. Do we ever think when we start a diet that this is something that we can do for the rest of our lives? Diets don't work because diet companies are trying to sell you a false promise that you believe and the only thing that it does is put money in their pockets. Diet companies are smart though; they know that you don't want to hear the truth. You want to keep on doing what you are doing because it instantly gratifies you and you like that. So you go for the diet that promises you that you don't have to give anything up and you can keep eating the things that you like (that presently are making you fat and sick) and it sells, in the billions.

Has it worked? In order to lose weight you need to confront the addictive, self-destructive behavior associated with the foods you eat and drinks you consume. Not too many people are willing to do that, so it is a tough thing to market as the latest and greatest diet fad. If you want to be successful in your weight-loss journey, your diet must consist of good nutrition that does not include animal products, olive oil or other fats, or processed or artificial foods. Permanent success is a lifestyle that incorporates 100% whole, plant-based foods.

Dr. Joel Fuhrman MD explains why diets don't work in Nutrient Density is the Key to Good Health (http://www.youtube.com/watch?v=XZGgeGHU1Bs).

How to Apply Plant Power

The idea is to add whole, plant-based foods to your diet that you don't already eat or get enough of and then start eliminating the foods and beverages that are making you fat and sick. If you know that you are having difficulty giving up certain foods, I recommend the monthly elimination approach. You can adjust when you choose to eliminate foods and beverages to biweekly or weekly as you see fit. Remember, elimination means elimination, not eating the food or drinking the beverage once in a while.

Read the food elimination chart on page 39. Check off any foods that you already have eliminated from your diet, or don't already eat. Choose how often you want to eliminate the foods and beverages from your diet; monthly, biweekly, weekly, or cold turkey. Refer to the "Foods to Eat" chapter on page 27 and the "Cooking Advice" chapter on page 79 to help you start making the right food choices.

Monthly

Eliminate one or more foods and beverages from your elimination chart once a month every month until you are eating 100% whole, plant-based food.

Biweekly

Eliminate one or more foods and beverages from your elimination chart once every two weeks until you are eating 100% whole, plant-based food.

Weekly

Eliminate one or more foods and beverages from your elimination chart once a week every week until you are eating 100% whole, plant-based food.

Cold Turkey

Eliminate all the items from the food elimination chart at once and only eat whole, plant-based foods listed throughout this book. Do a thorough house and kitchen cleaning by throwing out every food item that is not whole, plant-based food. Make a list and go shopping to restock your cupboards and refrigerator. Successfully using the cold turkey method can be difficult for some, but if you think that you can do it, that's fantastic. Let me know how it goes!

Foods to Eat

Carbohydrates are good for you; they are not the enemy of the person who needs to lose body fat. Just don't consume them from a can of cola or a processed snack. Carbohydrates are our energy source and they allow our brains to function. We also crave them, and they help to replenish us, give us energy, and fill us up. The carbohydrates you eat must come from food's most natural state with the nutrients and fiber still intact. This does not mean processed food, it means whole foods such as fruits, vegetables, grains, legumes, nuts, and seeds.

Protein is vital to our lives; it helps us function, grow, and live. The amount of protein you need is not what the media advertisers want you to believe. Remember, they are trying to sell you a product. The current theory is that you need 5-6% of your total calories per day from protein and maybe up to 9-10% for some athletes. If you eat a 2,000-calorie-per-day diet to maintain your present weight, the amount of protein needed is 25-30 grams (4 calories/gram) per day. Too much concentrated protein from animal sources will promote cancer growth and lead to other health issues such as high cholesterol.

Fat is misunderstood, and we eat way too much of it. People believe that olive oil is healthy when it is pure fat with no nutritional value. For survival purposes, we need to eat a minimum of 1-2 grams of fat per day. Most of your fat should come naturally from plant foods such as nuts and seeds. Walnuts are a good source of omega-3. (You would have to drink 8 ounces of olive oil to get the daily recommended amount of omega-3, which equals 1,900 calories.) There will always be some extra fats in your diet, but avoid adding it in by using salad dressings made with fat or cooking with oils and vegan butters.

Macronutrients are the foods we take in larger quantities, such as carbohydrates, proteins, fats, and water. Except for water, macronutrients contain calories. Micronutrients, such as vitamins, minerals, and disease-fighting phytochemicals, keep our bodies and brains healthy by nourishing us and help us fight off diseases such as cancer and Alzheimer's disease. These are taken in small quantities, contain no calories, and are abundantly found in organic, unprocessed plant foods. When you live on a processed food diet, you can become malnourished from not getting enough micronutrients. When your body doesn't receive its required micronutrients from whole food sources, it sends hunger signals out to get more food. As a result, we keep eating more and more micronutrient-deficient macronutrients, which makes us feel terrible, zapping our energy, and we gain more weight. Try to eat at least 20 different varieties of fruits, vegetables, and legumes daily, including some nuts, seeds, and grains.

Eat sugar and salt. What? Yes, it is important to have a little sugar and salt in your diet every day. Our taste buds on our tongues seek the tastes of sugar and salt, which is one reason we are so easily addicted to sugary and salted foods. The fast-food industries capitalize on this. Trying to completely deprive yourself of either sugar or salt will eventually lead to a meltdown, and you might find yourself wolfing down an entire bag of chemically made, trans fat, cream-filled chocolate sandwich cookies, or munching mindlessly on your friend's french fry order. A little goes a long way, so take in just enough sugar and salt to be satisfied. Try lightly salting your homemade soup just before you eat it and adding a little maple syrup to your oatmeal for breakfast. That's it. Pay attention to the salt and sugar content of your food and, as always, try to avoid all processed foods.

How many calories should you get every day? This is tough to tell you exactly because there are so many variables that play into your caloric expenditure. Your age, sex, weight, and physical activity are just a few. If you are not active and don't exercise, you'd be surprised at how few calories you burn. For example, if you are a 40-year-old female who weighs 160 pounds and doesn't do any physical activity, you probably need only 1,400-1,500 calories a day. Some people get more than that just from the beverages that they consume. The best thing to do is to add exercise to your life and stick to your balanced whole, plant-based diet. Exercise increases your caloric expenditure, and a plant-based diet will give you more food for your calories. Your body will feel satisfied not just from the quantity, but from the nutrient density of the food, and naturally you won't want to overeat.

Be careful of your wheat intake, because many of us have wheat intolerances and we don't even know it. When you adopt a whole, plant-based diet, wheat products such as yummy whole-grain breads can become too much of a staple food. Eat whole-grain breads sparingly or not at all because they are very dense and can add a lot of extra calories to your diet. Also too much wheat (and sometimes rice) can bloat and constipate you. If you find that you are bloated, gassy, fatigued, or lack energy, lay off some grains, including wheat, barley, oats, and rye products, to see if that helps.

For more information on foods to eat, I recommend: Understanding Calorie Density with Jeff Novick, RD (http://www.youtube.com/watch?v=9gTLpTq1nQk).

Your Primary Food Sources

Try to eat at least one pound per day of the following:
- Green vegetables
- Edible raw vegetables
- Non-starchy cooked vegetables
- Fresh-picked or frozen fruit.

Also try to consume one cup per day of low- or no-salt beans and lentils.

These are your most nutrient-rich food sources, especially leafy green vegetables. It is important to eat a variety of vegetables and fruits, which you can do by choosing many different colored foods. This offers a synergistic effect of your proteins, vitamins, minerals, and phytochemicals (disease-fighting chemicals only found in non-processed plant foods).

Eat Enough to Meet Your Caloric Intake Needs

These are the food sources that you need to watch the quantity of to adjust your calories to lose, maintain, or gain weight:
- Cooked starchy vegetables such as potatoes, brown rice, and whole grains
- Unsalted nuts and seeds
- Avocados.

Beverages

When you are trying to lose weight, do not drink your calories! Instead, try these beverages:
- Water
- Herbal tea with no artificial flavoring

- Unflavored seltzer or club soda (add your own flavoring like fresh lemon or lime juice).

Eat These Rarely or Preferably Never (See Food Elimination Chart)

Foods to avoid or eliminate include the following:
- Meat, fish, dairy, and all animal products
- Processed food
- Fast food
- Oils and added fats
- Processed white sugar, white flour, and white rice
- High-sodium foods
- All soft drinks, diet drinks, energy drinks, juice drinks, coffee, and caffeinated beverages.

It is impossible to be perfect all the time, especially if you get caught off guard and you are in a situation where you need to eat and there is nothing healthy available at your present location. Just do the best you can. This is why it is important to plan ahead and be prepared. If you know that you are going to be in a situation where the only food available is pizza and wings, either eat beforehand or bring your own food. It might seem like a hassle, but it is worth it! There are a lot more people who do this than you realize, especially people with food allergies or food intolerances. They just keep it quiet to avoid hassles and judgments sometimes encountered from others.

Supplements

There is a lot of controversy over supplements. Most of the information we get about supplements comes from the companies that produce them. Unfortunately we really don't know what is exactly in these products and how they are made. Most supplements either don't work or can potentially do more damage than good. A popular myth is that protein powders build muscle tissue, which is not true. Using the muscle promotes muscle growth, and the protein you get naturally from whole-plant food sources is enough to support that growth. If you don't believe me, ask an elephant what he eats to maintain all that muscle mass!

A vitamin supplement is designed for the person who doesn't eat right, and taking too many vitamin and mineral supplements can have damaging and toxic effects. The best place to get your vitamins and minerals is from the variety of food sources you eat. Deficiencies on a plant-based diet could be vitamin D (not enough sunlight), or vitamin B12 (not readily available because our food sources are too clean), but the only way to know this is to get a blood test from a competent healthcare provider. The test will show you what and how much you are lacking and how much to supplement (not replace) your already healthy diet. Do not self-diagnose.

Calcium is a concern for women, especially as we age, but there are a lot of misunderstandings about calcium intake. The fear that we have is, if we don't drink enough milk we will get osteoporosis as we get older. The truth is that if we don't exercise enough it will age our bones, and mega dosing on calcium products won't reverse this. Dairy products have never been proven to have a positive effect on bone density. It may be necessary for you to take a calcium supplement, but it is important to first eliminate sources that can be stripping calcium from your body such as animal products, excessive salt, smoking, and caffeine. One of the best sources of calcium is green leafy vegetables, the same place the cow gets her calcium from.

For more interesting information on animal products and type I diabetes watch: Dr. McDougall's Type I Diabetes Caused by Milk (http://www.vegsource.com/news/2011/05/dr-mcdougall-type-1-diabetes-caused-by-milk-video.html).

Read Food Labels

If you can't pronounce it or you don't know what it is, don't buy it until you research it. Eliminating processed and unhealthy foods will allow you to greatly reduce the cost of your grocery bills. Remember the following:
- No enriched flours
- No trans (hydrogenated) fat
- No corn syrup or added processed sugar
- Low salt/sodium per serving should not exceed the calories per serving
- No artificial anything, including "natural flavors"
- No preservatives and no MSG.

Jeff Novick, RD explains some of the food labels and how they are misleading. Watch How to Read Food Labels (http://www.youtube.com/watch?v=yd9XnyNGXGs) and When Fat Free Really Means 100% Fat (http://www.youtube.com/watch?feature=player_embedded&v=1pD3-j0GdWo).

Food Elimination Chart

Food/Beverage	Date of Elimination from Diet
Cheese	
Milk/yogurt/other dairy products	
Ice cream	
Fish	
Beef	
Pork	
Chicken	
Fried food	
Fast food	
Pizza (unhealthy version)	
Candy	
Soda pop, including diet	
Energy drinks	
Beer	
Wine/liquor	
Fruit juice/juice drinks	
Cookies/crackers/chips	
Unhealthy desserts	
Eggs	
Chocolate	
Butter	
Mayo	
Caffeine	
Sugar/white flour/white rice	
Oil/fat	
Other:	

Explanation of the Food Elimination Chart

After reading the food elimination chart, are you shocked that you have to give all that stuff up? It is shocking that you put all those energy-sucking, cancer-causing, heart disease-inducing substances into your body in the first place. If your food comes from anything processed, including animal products, you are putting yourself at risk for being overweight and, worse yet, acquiring obesity-related health issues such as impotence, diabetes, stroke, and heart disease.

Eliminating unhealthy foods not just from your diet, but from your grocery list and from your house, is important. Buying a bag of candy as a treat for the kids is not only unhealthy and unnecessary, but it is lying to yourself. If you have a weight problem, you have an addiction problem. You know that if it is in your house, it will be in your mouth. Only stock your kitchen with healthy, whole, plant-based foods.

Listed on the following pages is a brief overview of why you need to eliminate these foods from your body permanently.

Meat, Fish and Eggs

Animal fat and proteins are the cause of many illnesses, such as but not limited to: heart disease, cancers (liver, breast, prostate, colon, pancreas, etc.), obesity, gallstones, kidney stones, Alzheimer's disease, dementia, behavior and mood disorders, osteoporosis, infantile iron deficiency anemia, cataracts, and diarrhea/dysentery.

Animal products are high in saturated fats, have cholesterol, and may contain e-coli. Animal products contain antibiotics, steroids, manure, growth hormones, and pesticides (pesticides found in animal products can be 13 times the amount found in plant foods). Animal products don't contain antioxidants or phytochemicals and are very high in calories.

Deli meat contains nitrates, which are considered to be carcinogens (cancer-causing substances). When combined with the animal proteins and saturated fat, this could never be healthy.

Fish are polluted from the waste we pollute all our water systems with, such as fertilizers, pesticides, sewage, and oil spills. Pregnant women, nursing women, and young children should never eat fish because it causes brain damage from the mercury contamination.

Eggs have the sulfur-containing amino acid methionine, which is metabolized into homocysteine. This causes risk factors associated with heart attacks, strokes, peripheral vascular disease, Alzheimer's disease, and depression.

Meat and dairy production is the single biggest contributor to global warming. A Prius-driving meat eater contributes to more gas emissions then a vegan-eating Hummer driver. Imagine a meat-eating Hummer driver!

For more information, read the McDougall Newsletter Vol. 4 No. 3 for more information on eggs.
(http://drmcdougall.com/misc/2005nl/march/050300pueastereggs.htm).
Also read John Robbins How To Win An Argument With A Meat Eater (http://www.vegsource.com/news/2009/09/how-to-win-an-argument-with-a-meat-eater.html).

Dairy

We are not meant to drink milk after we are weaned. What do most animals drink after they are weaned? Yes, water.

We are not designed to drink another species' milk. You might ask, what about my calcium? Your calcium should mostly come from plant sources such as green leafy vegetables, the same place that many large muscle-bearing animals such as horses or gorillas get their calcium from. Dairy products are high in cholesterol and saturated fat. They can also be contaminated with disease-causing, nonfood-like substances such as pesticides, growth hormones, manure, antibiotics, and steroids. Dairy products are also known to enhance skin problems such as acne and can intensify your allergies.

Cheese is 70%-90% fat, seriously! Yogurt can be high in sugar with no fiber, or worse, aspartame (a brain damaging chemical sweetener). Yogurt is not a health food.

Positive health information related to dairy products comes from resources such as the American Dairy Association and Dairy Counsel, which is not based on long-term scientific studies but is contrived for marketing purposes solely for profit with no actual concern for your health.

T. Colin Campbell's Animal Protein-Meat and Dairy Cause Cancer (http://www.youtube.com/watch?v=yfsT-qYeGqM).

Fast Food, Fried Food, and Pizza

Fast food is a death sentence, and it should be classified as child abuse if you get your kids hooked on it. It is chemically processed; loaded with saturated fat, hydrogenated, or trans fat (really bad); very high in sodium; low in nutrients; and extremely addictive.

Chicken nuggets are made from all parts of mechanically separated chickens that are turned into a paste and then processed and fried into something so gross! This is called "advanced meat recovery" and is found in processed meats. Fast-food ground beef (pink slime) is washed in ammonia (a highly poisonous substance) to kill e-coli. Yum!

Fried food has little nutrient density and excessive calories and fat. Pizza in the traditional sense is junk food, but it can be reworked into something healthy by eliminating the animal products and using whole grains and vegetables.

Processed fast food kills more people than all the terrorism in the world.

I recommend watching the Supersize Me documentary (http://www.youtube.com/watch?v=I1Lkyb6SU5U) and to read more on how fast food is really made: (http://

www.vegsource.com/news/2010/10/this-is-what-chicken-mcnuggets-looks-like----seriously.html).

Candy, Cookies, and Unhealthy Desserts

First of all, these are just fattening and addictive. They are loaded with chemicals, nonfood-like substances, sugar, saturated fat, and animal products. Unhealthy desserts should never be eaten, and healthy desserts should be avoided while trying to lose weight, especially if you are not active and don't get any exercise.

Soda, Energy Drinks, Fruit Juice, and Juice Drinks

Soda, aka: obesity pop. It has no nutritional value, and let's face it, it's a sugar addict's fix. If it's the bubbles you like, drink seltzer water with fresh lemon or lime.

Energy drinks are highly caffeinated and loaded with stimulants that mess with your blood pressure. They dehydrate you and make your blood sugar spike, and then you crash, which inevitably makes you nonproductive. They contribute to and enhance mood and behavior disorders. Since energy drinks are relatively new on the market, long-term effects have yet to be determined.

Diet sodas and other sugar-free drinks are usually chemically sweetened with aspartame, which has been associated with several types of cancer.

Fruit juice is high in calories. It is stripped of its fiber and we tend to consume more than the recommended serving size. Fresh or frozen fruit is always better. Juice drinks and juice boxes are artificially processed and sometimes produced in countries that have no sanitation laws for the water used to produce these drinks.

For more information on aspartame, watch Aspartame, NutraSweet, Artificial Sweetener & Diet Soda (http://www.youtube.com/watch?v=TgKbD_QClxA).

Alcohol

Alcohol makes you stupid. It makes you do and say stupid things. It also makes you fat, unless you drink so much that it makes you sick when you eat. Then you look really sick and really stupid. It causes liver damage, brain damage, cancer, and decreased productivity levels; destroys your memory; gives you terrible hangovers; and can disrupt your sleep. Unfortunately alcohol is socially acceptable in our culture and we are very unaware of the actual amount of alcoholism that surrounds us.

Alcohol is a known carcinogen that can increase the risk of breast cancer. It is not part of a healthy diet and it will sabotage all your good work toward feeling good and losing weight.

Read more about alcohol and increased cancer risk with Jeff Novick, RD
(http://www.vegsource.com/talk/novick/messages/1041.html).

Sugar

Sugar is highly addictive, and the withdrawal symptoms when you don't eat sugar are equivalent to what a heroin addict goes through. White flour (stripped of its fiber and nutrients) works in your bloodstream like sugar. It raises your blood sugar levels quickly, which makes you feel really good until your blood sugar levels drop. Then your body starts to crash and detox, and then you don't feel so good. So again, you reach for the white stuff. Suddenly you feel better, and the cycle repeats. The results: you gain weight and suffer the consequences and illnesses of being overweight such as obesity, diabetes, stroke, cardiovascular disease, Alzheimer's disease, tooth decay, and macular degeneration (loss of vision). Too much sugar is also blamed for causing premature aging, like wrinkles.

Because we all crave sugar in some form and it is a source of energy, it is very difficult to eliminate it from your diet. You must be smart about how you get your sugar and not overindulge. I will increase my sugar intake (from whole food sources like fruits) if I know that I am going to burn off more than 1,000 extra calories in a day. Otherwise I stick to having my daily sugar fix with my breakfast oatmeal or quinoa with a variety of fruits and a tablespoon of maple syrup.

Read this great article titled Sugar is Poison, provided by vegsource.com (http://www.vegsource.com/news/2011/04/sugar-is-a-poison-says-ucsf-obesity-expert.html).

Caffeine

Caffeine is addictive and it comes in many forms such as some sodas, coffee, and energy drinks. Here are a few reasons why you shouldn't drink it: it increases blood pressure, nervousness, irritability, dehydration, menstrual pain, insomnia, headaches, Alzheimer's disease, irregular heartbeat, muscle tremors, and anxiety, and can deplete calcium from your bones.

Coffee is made from coffee beans that are usually imported and sprayed with pesticides that have been banned in this country. For the USDA to actually ban something, you know it must be really bad. Coffee stains your teeth, which will make you look old. It is also believed that cancer cells love to feed off the acid produced in your body from coffee.

Oil and Fat

Fat and oil have no nutritional value, so for the most part the fat you eat is the fat you wear. It's important to pay attention to the amount of fat that is in your food, especially from processed and restaurant foods. There are nine calories per gram of fat, and that can add up very quickly.

Sodium

Sodium or salt is a necessary nutrient. We crave it, and it brings out the flavors in our food. A healthy amount of salt per day is less than a teaspoon. Too much salt can contribute to high blood pressure and heart disease. It also deadens your ability to taste food without salt. This is why when you remove salt from your diet, your food will taste very bland and almost unpalatable. Getting used to the taste of foods without or with very little added salt takes a little bit of time.

Health Foods

Not all health foods are created equal. Beware of imitation meats and cheese. Just because a product is labeled vegan, dairy free, or organic does not mean that it is healthy. Read the labels and check for high fat, salt, sugar, and processed and artificial ingredients.

Problems That You Can Run Into When You Are Trying to Lose Weight

One of the biggest issues that sabotages weight loss is not knowing how to deal with and work through the problems that arise. Your problems need to be challenged, overcome, learned from, and not used as an excuse to give up.

Belief System

Everyone has a belief system; it is how we function (emotionally and behaviorally) in our lives. Our belief systems are developed starting when we are born from our upbringing and from the environment in which we live. It's what we know that we believe works, right or wrong, and when what we believe is wrong, it is very difficult to change even if we know better. Usually major changes that we make in our lives are based on how we feel and not just on what we know. You can read every book written on plant-based lifestyles, but if it is too drastic a change from what you have always believed, it can be way too difficult for some to emotionally manage or even contemplate.

Plant-based lifestyles are nothing new; they have been around since the beginning of man and are still prominent in many cultures. Vegetarian, vegan, and plant-based lifestyles are growing in popularity in this country. We are hearing more about it in the media and many businesses are capitalizing on it, especially in some food industries, farming, and healthier restaurants (usually found in larger cities). It will take time for it to be accepted as part of our society's belief system, probably generations away, but for now it is important to believe that if you live on our present culturally accepted foods, you will end up sick and you will eventually pay the price.

Addiction

Addiction is a coping method. Addiction is a denial that what you are doing to yourself is physically and psychologically unhealthy, and self-destructive. We all do it. It could be anything from taking drugs, smoking, or drinking, to eating junk food. We know it's bad, but we still do it. We ignore the consequences of our actions, such as pain, fatigue, and long-term chronic disease. We teach our bad habits to our children. Most of all, when someone points out our addictions we don't want to hear it! We always rationalize what we do wrong and tend to socialize with others like us for protection from the truth. We even look for justifications, especially for our food addictions, which are readily found in the media due to the billions of dollars that are spent every year by advertisers to help us keep our addictions.

To manage your addictions, you need to replace the addiction with another coping method. What can you do that makes you feel good and isn't unhealthy? Some people turn to athletics, hobbies, meditating, or helping others. It is important to find something that you are passionate about. It should make you feel good when you do it, and it shouldn't come with adverse side effects.

Eliminating unhealthy food addictions is not something most people are willing to do. Many people don't realize that they have food addictions, while others have been told but are in denial. Most people are not well educated about nutrition and how it affects just about every aspect of our lives. Food addiction is a serious epidemic that is not being focused on enough by healthcare providers and appropriate governmental agencies.

Withdrawal

You must come to terms with your addictions by admitting that you have them. You must decide to eliminate your addictions and have a real inner driving goal or reason for doing so. Here comes the hard part; managing the detoxification and the withdrawal effects. The intensity of the discomfort from the detox associated with giving up certain foods such as excessive sugar, salt, and caffeine varies from person to person. It can bring on such symptoms as physical discomfort, anxiety, anger, rage, and stress, which is where the majority of us fail and regain our previous addictions.

Going through withdrawal is part of the process of getting healthy and losing weight. It takes time and it will not be easy, but it can be done if the desire to do so is strong. Some people can find it too daunting to accomplish by themselves; if this is the case, it is important to seek help from a plant-based weight loss professional.

For more information on nutritional counseling, contact Nunda Nutritional Counseling, LLC (www.nundanutrition.com).

Exercise

When you are starting to exercise and you don't normally exercise or you just hate it, it can be very difficult to stay motivated. If you are overweight, it is especially hard because it hurts, and it's embarrassing to have people watch you. I really didn't like people seeing my fat butt running down the road in shorts that I should never wear in public, so I headed to the woods and did trail running. This might not work in your situation, but it is important to find reasons or personal motivations (not excuses) to exercise every day. Look at it this way; never exercising is to your body like what happens to your teeth if you never brush them. Exercising is difficult when you are overweight, so it is very important to eat only plant-based foods to help you stay feeling good and keep you from losing motivation.

Cravings

Cravings can attack at any time. This is part of the addiction and withdrawal process. Here are some ways to deal with your cravings:

Hunger: If you are hungry, eat. Eat fruit or vegetables. Hunger is only manageable when you eat nutrient-dense foods.

Sugar: Need a sugar fix? Eat fresh seasonal or frozen fruit. It has the sugar you are craving but it also comes with a dose of fiber and nutrients. This will help keep your blood sugar from spiking and will save you from the inevitable crash later. Try my hot fruit recipe on page 117.

Salt: It takes time (months) for your body to adapt to the flavors of unsalted, whole, plant-based foods, so you must be patient with this. Always taste your food before salting it and add just a scant amount to bring out the natural flavors of your foods.

Don't keep junk food in the house: This can be tough when you live with unhealthy family members or you don't do the shopping, but if possible don't keep any unhealthy foods in your house, because you know that if they are there, you will most likely eat them.

Indulgences: Are you going to be perfect and never eat anything that is bad for you for the rest of your life? Probably not, but the best way to manage indulgences and not get off track on your healthy eating is to plan for your indulgences. I have been eating a plant-based diet long enough that I really don't crave bad foods very much. I also get repulsed by the idea of putting high amounts of fat and chemicals into my body, but my one indulgence that I plan for is chocolate on Christmas. Each Christmas, I allow myself to eat dairy-free chocolate, usually from a really good chocolate shop. I spend too much and I eat as much of it as I feel like, because I planned for it. I look forward to it, I don't feel guilty about eating it, and because it happens only once a year, it doesn't affect my weight.

Stress

Stress is always a part of life. Sometimes it is worse than usual and sometimes it seems almost unbearable. Unfortunately stress can be used as an excuse to eat unhealthy food. "I have so much stress in my life, I just can't take on something new right now." This statement usually gets a lot of sympathy from friends and family, which can be very comforting, but it is self-destructive. Stress never completely goes away from our lives, and being unhealthy and overweight will cause a lot of your stress.

Remember that when things seem really terrible in your life, it helps to be grateful for what you have by making a mental list of what you are blessed with and practicing being thankful for these blessings. For example, I am grateful for my warm home, my kids, my intelligence, my talents, and this beautiful day. Another way to manage stress is to do something nice for someone else, because helping somebody who is less fortunate or having difficulties can put things in perspective and will always make you feel better!

The Scale

Avoid it. Weighing yourself on a regular basis can be psychologically and emotionally damaging. Your weight will fluctuate throughout the day and throughout the week. This is usually due to water intake and expenditure, and seeing a one- or two-pound fluctuation can sabotage your motivation. The most often you should check your weight is once a month, but preferably twice a year just out of curiosity. Let your clothes tell the truth. If you're going down in pants sizes, it's working!

The Dreaded Plateau

If you have ever been on a diet, you know what the plateau is. It is when you think that you are doing all the right things but you aren't losing any weight. There are a few things that you can do to overcome this.

First, reevaluate your diet. Even if you are eating 100% whole, plant-based food, you could still be overdoing it in the calorie department. Are you eating too many sweets? Are you eating too many starchy foods, such as wheat products? Watch your calories for a few days and see if some trimming is necessary. Also make sure that you are getting enough calories. If you are not eating enough, you will feel weak and not be able to exercise. This can result in loss of muscle and metabolic slow down.

Second, how is your exercise routine? Are you putting in as much as you can? Maybe you need to change things up, change your routine, or buy some different workout videos. Changing your exercise routine is good, because it can keep you motivated. Also watch out for overtraining, which can result in fatigue, burnout, and injury.

Most of all, be patient, because your body needs time to adjust. Remember, this is a lifestyle change, not a temporary fix.

Clothing Expense

This might be a good problem to have! You've lost weight and now your clothes don't fit. Most people have some clothes in their closet that used to be too small that now fit, and what a reward! Realistically if you don't have any clothes that fit, and your budget is a concern, shop at Goodwill or places like it. It is very trendy and green right now to shop at secondhand stores. Drop off your "fat clothes" and buy some new-to-you "skinny clothes." This saves you a lot of money, especially if you are still going down a few more sizes. Don't turn your nose up at secondhand clothes. You'll find some great stuff there, and you'll be helping the environment and contributing to a charitable cause.

Doctors and Their Prescription Pads

It amazes me that one can go to one's doctor and within five minutes of one's conversation with him or her, the doctor is already writing a prescription. "Take this two times a day and call me in six months."

When I was 29, I went to a specialist because I was having severe issues with anxiety from PMS. He wrote me a prescription for Prozac. He said, "Take this and you will start to feel better in three weeks." He got up and walked out of the room. This took less than five minutes, and I spent twenty minutes in the waiting room. I sat there for a moment, dumbfounded. To think that I was expecting an explanation of why. I left that office with no answers to my unasked questions, a little bit poorer and a lot more confused. Not knowing any better, I did what he said. I took the pills because I thought they would cure me. Was I wrong! After a few weeks, I was in a continual state of fog, I had no ambition and no sex drive, and I found that camping out on my couch was about all I could do. I finally smartened up and stopped taking the drug, although he told me not to do so without his permission. Why would I want another appointment with someone who put me on this life-sucking drug? It took me another month to get this chemical garbage out of my system and snap out of it. I decided to figure out what I could do on my own to solve my problem. It took me a long time to figure this out, but changing my diet, staying active, and practicing a balanced lifestyle proved to be the most effective and inexpensive prescription.

A few years ago, I was talking to a doctor outside of the medical office environment, and the conversation was mainly about the business end of his medical profession. He said that in order for his practice to be profitable he needed to see 24 patients per day, about four patients per hour. How on earth can you conscientiously make medical decisions on behalf of another human being in 15 minutes or less? It takes me longer to pick out a pair of shoes.

Most pills that doctors prescribe for weight-related issues such as diabetes and heart disease do not cure you. They maintain you where you are at and add negative side effects on top of all your problems. Make sure your doctor talks to you, listens to you, and gives you all of your options. Make sure that your doctor is discussing the underlying causes of your illnesses and not just treating the symptoms with profit-making pharmaceuticals. If not, find another doctor. There are a few good ones out there, it just seems hard to find one.

Ridicule

Being ridiculed about making healthy lifestyle choices is probably one of the most difficult challenges that you will have to face. You will be amazed at what people say in their own defense to rationalize their own unhealthy lifestyle. You might be insulted and belittled, and the saddest thing is that most of the ridicule usually comes from your close friends and family.

When people give you a hard time about living healthfully, it can be hurtful and you will want to lash back, but you need to realize where it is coming from. It is not about you, it is the attackers' way of defending themselves. Deep down inside they know you are right, but your lifestyle is a constant reminder of how fat and unhealthy they really are. Their belief system is challenged, and they won't allow themselves to face that. The best thing to do when someone attacks your nutritional and lifestyle-related changes is to not respond at all. I found this out the hard way. I suggested in an indirect way to someone who I thought was a friend that he might have sugar addiction issues (he had asked for weight-loss advice). He flipped and proceeded to verbally attack me, calling me a born-again vegan, and now he avoids me like the plague. It bothered me at first, but I have to remember that it's not about me, but about how he really feels about himself. People will feel threatened by you all the time just because you are taking steps to be healthy. So prepare yourself for the unbelievable comments and attacks, keep your comments to yourself, and let it go! Be true to yourself, and hopefully the ones who love you the most will support you and maybe even join you.

Second-guessing Yourself

There are times, especially in social situations, that you will start to second-guess yourself and the changes that you have made. We are constantly bombarded with food, from TV, magazines, parties, meetings, family gatherings, etcetera. If you are the only one you know who lives a plant-powered lifestyle, it can make you feel like you are out of the "club" and a little alienated. Look to your goals or original reason for getting healthy and losing weight and use that as your strength and empowerment. It's about what is right for you, not about what other people think.

There are also good memories associated with food, such as "My Mom made the best macaroni and cheese," or when you smell someone grilling out and it smells so good. After a while when you've been exclusively plant-based, you realize that it's actually the comfort of the memories you miss. Thinking about eating grilled animal flesh and artery-clogging cheese will eventually gross you out. If you do eat the bad stuff, it won't taste as good as you might have remembered and can make you feel very sick.

When you are making your best effort to eat and live healthfully, you will make a bigger impact than you realize. By not eating meat you are reducing your carbon footprint, reducing profit margins for junk food companies, and influencing people around you, even if you only make them second-guess what they are putting into their bodies. Good for you!

Be strong and tell yourself that you are doing the right thing, not necessarily the easy thing.

Excuses

Sometimes I think that I have heard every lame excuse, but if I haven't I can hear one coming from a mile away! Imagine the following conversation:

Me: "No thank you, I don't eat dairy."

My friend: "You don't eat dairy, then what do you eat?

Me: "My doctor told me to lose weight because my cholesterol is 220."

My friend: "So how did you lose all that weight?"

Me: "I stopped eating dairy." My friend is still looking at me in confusion.

My friend: "Well, I could never give up my cheese!"

This conversation happens to me more often than you might think. For some people it's cheese and for others it's meat, sugar, or beer. Think about it. Are you being controlled by your food or are you in denial? Do you live to eat or eat to live?

"I've tried everything." Now tell me what unhealthy foods you refuse to give up.

"I don't like the taste of water." You don't like the taste of water because it is not loaded with sugar and cola flavored.

"Wine is good for you. It has antioxidants." Wine is alcohol and extra calories. Get your antioxidants from non-fermented fruit and vegetables.

"My husband keeps bringing fast food home for dinner." Is he holding a gun to your head and forcing you to eat it? Be stronger and smarter than him and stand your ground.

"I have a slow metabolism." A slow metabolism helps keep you from prematurely aging. It's total energy expenditure that you need to increase and bad food you need to decrease. You could be in denial about what and how much you actually eat and if you don't exercise on top of that, what do you expect?

"I have bad genes." If you are genetically predisposed to certain diseases, then you would think that you would be especially careful about any disease-causing foods that you would put into your body (genes can't act alone). Otherwise you are using this excuse to play the victim.

We all rationalize why we eat what we eat. Many times we are eating foods we think are healthy because some doctor on TV said they were. Doctors on TV get paid and are scripted on what to say. TV stations are owned by or tied directly with the major food corporations, and their job is to sell you a product to make money. We like hearing that the unhealthful food we eat is good for us so we can keep eating it, stay sick, and wonder why we can't lose weight! Read the fine print on those doctors' websites and it will say things like, "For entertainment purposes only."

Challenge yourself by challenging your excuses. The biggest lies that we repeatedly tell ourselves are about our weight and our health. It's not easy to confront your excuses and make changes. It takes character and self-esteem. You can make the changes needed to get healthy!

Relapse

Relapses happen. It's what you do about it that counts. Some people use a relapse as an excuse to give up, saying "Oh, I can't stick to anything." This is not an option. Screwing up is a part of life and it should be viewed as an opportunity to do better. Let's say that you went out with some friends and had a couple of glasses of wine, got a little drunk, and then devoured a whole plate of cheese nachos. Hopefully you will feel terrible the next day as a reminder of how toxic junk can be to your body. Then reevaluate the situation that put you there in the first place. What was your mood? What made you drink and eat what you did? What will you do differently next time? Maybe order club soda and something healthy to eat. Maybe avoid the environment or people that put you in an unhealthy situation. Figure it out for yourself, revisit your goal for getting healthy, and make the necessary changes so it doesn't happen again.

Hormones

If you are female, you know what hormones can do to your appetite. Eating a plant-based diet and eliminating the junk and caffeine can help a great deal if you suffer from PMS or menopausal symptoms. It will reduce some of the discomfort, pain, anxiety, and hunger.

If you are using a form of birth control, this can make it difficult to lose weight. It can make your body feel like it's pregnant, which can make you want to eat constantly or too much at one time. Unfortunately taking birth control sometimes has to be a part of our lives, and the best way to manage overeating is to avoid calorie-dense foods and stick to nutrient-dense, plant-based foods.

Balance

To stay mentally and physically fit and enjoy life the best you can, it is important to have a sense of balance in your life. When you have balance, you can develop good health, which leads to permanent weight loss.
Listed below are some ways to attain balance. Balancing your life takes desire, commitment, education, and practice.

Nutrition
Good nutrition is the best medicine. If you eat right you will feel right. Good nutrition is one of the most important things that you can do for your health, so don't underestimate its power.

Exercise
Your body is designed to move. You must move to be healthy and prevent illness. Yoga is a good way to gain flexibility, prevent injury, and feel better. Strength training and aerobic exercise also add to a balanced physical state.

Mindfulness
Pay attention to what you do. Are you doing the right thing? Pay attention to the food that you put

in your mouth and why you are eating it. Pay attention to what you say and how it affects other people. Be mindful.

Gratefulness
Gratefulness should be practiced on a daily basis. If you think that you have it bad, I promise you someone else has it worse. Being grateful for who you are and what you have helps reduce stress and allows you to be happy. If you don't like your situation, do what you can to change it and be grateful that you have the strength to do so.

Education
Continual learning keeps our minds sharp and healthy as we age. Read or learn how to do something new no matter how young or old you are.

Spirituality
Spirituality can help you find inner peace by becoming more compassionate and selfless. It can also help you develop sustainable, healthy values.

Meditation
Meditation helps de-stress your mind and body. You learn to train your mind to replace many

thoughts with just one. Meditation takes guidance and practice.

Random Acts of Kindness
When you perform a random act of kindness, such as helping someone you don't know, without expecting anything in return, not only have you brought a little comfort into someone else's life but it can be one of the most rewarding things that you ever experience.

Family
Time is one of the most important things that you can give your family. The quality of your time is defined by simple things such as listening and showing interest. Practice this with your loved ones every day.

Self-esteem
How do you feel about yourself? If you don't like who you are, make changes. If you don't think you are good enough, smart enough, or attractive enough, you are wrong. Successful people come from all walks of life and have all different backgrounds. Don't make excuses for what you are doing or not doing, especially when you know you are doing the right thing. Don't allow a bad past to

negatively define your future. Take pride and comfort in following your own path.

Social Activities
Don't miss out on life because you have low self-esteem. Get out and live your life, enjoy the good, and let go of the bad. Look for the good things in your friends and colleagues, be less judgmental, and avoid gossiping. Show up in life, experience the good and the bad, and it will pay off.

Motivation
Self-motivation can make life productive and meaningful. Start with something simple like dressing your best for the situation, even if you are just working around the house or going to buy groceries. (Please don't wear pajamas and sweats in public!) Act like you are worth a billion dollars and take pride in the simplest of things, such as how nice of a job you have done in the most menial of situations like cleaning a bathroom or sweeping the floor.

Manners
Manners are a lost art these days. I find when I am in a busy place people don't say something as simple as "excuse me" when they are trying to get

by me. Lead by example because it's not just the young people who are rude, it's people of all ages. Practicing good manners and common courtesies help people live together peacefully.

Sleep
Turn off the TV and go to bed. Get eight or nine hours of sleep each night. If you have a hard time sleeping, pay attention to the lack of balance in your life because being out of balance (especially due to poor nutrition) will affect all aspects of your sleep.

Positive Thoughts
When negative thoughts are invading your mind, stop them in their tracks and change gears. Focus on something good or positive and stay with it until you feel the tension in your body release. Avoid making excuses for the things that you do and don't follow someone else's path. You know when you are doing the right thing.

Don't stop here. What brings value to your life? When you are always striving to learn and to be a better person, you will find the balance and satisfaction in your life. It will also allow you to set and achieve goals such as weight loss and good health.

Cooking Advice

I am a lazy, unmotivated cook, but I do know how important it is to make my own meals and eat the healthiest foods possible. If you are a gourmet cook or cooking is your hobby, there are thousands of recipes that you can find on the Internet and there are more whole, plant-based cookbooks being published all the time. Just beware of some vegan and vegetarian recipes, because they tend to use a lot of fat and processed, refined foods.

The recipes in this book are simple, call for commonly available ingredients, and are good on a budget. When you cook, always make enough for leftovers so you can save them for lunch the next day or freeze them for when you don't have time to shop or cook. Another option is to cook for the week, especially soups and stews. It takes me about 15 minutes to prepare a full crock pot of soup. I let the soup cook all day or night in the crock pot on low and then put it in freezer containers (after it cools) to have individual servings for later.

Start a Garden

Even if you haven't ever gardened before, there is something amazing about going to your garden to get fresh ingredients for your dinner. Potatoes, carrots, Swiss chard, tomatoes, onions, garlic, herbs, and peppers are just some of the things that you can grow. If you don't have any land, try container gardening. I do both. That way, when it gets cold in the fall I can bring my potted herbs, tomatoes, and peppers indoors to keep warm. If you don't have much room or are a first-time gardener, start small with a few herb plants like basil, oregano, and parsley. Gardening is one of the world's most popular hobbies, and your results get you the freshest and most nutrient-rich, organic, non-GMO and pesticide-free food available. There are plenty of gardening resources online, in books, in the media, and from community gardening classes. Keep it organic and make gardening a family project.

Don't forget to compost! Save all of your vegetable and fruit scraps and compost them. Add leaves and any organic matter to make your own nutrient-rich dirt. Add your seasoned dirt to your garden, to keep your plants coming back strong and high yielding every year.

Get Your Kids Involved in Cooking

What are your kids doing while you are preparing dinner, their homework? If they are, good for them, but most likely they are attached to some electronic device. Not a good idea!

There are so many reasons for cooking with your kids. It teaches them safety, responsibility, and a needed skill. It will give you quality time with your kids and it might even give them some appreciation for what you do.

You don't have to be a good cook. Kids are creative and will help you out with new ideas. Encourage this even though you know cocoa powder might not taste so good in the tomato soup. Teach your kids all aspects of cooking, starting with the planning, shopping, preparing, cooking, and cleaning up. Your meals will be more enjoyable and less rushed. Your kids will eat a wider variety of food because they made it themselves. If you can, start them cooking while they are young because by the time they are teenagers they should be preparing your meals. Then they have earned the right to play with their electronic devices!

Eating Out

Good luck! Maybe you live in an area that offers vegetarian or vegan cuisine. It is definitely starting to grow in popularity. If you live in a rural area like I do, it is almost impossible to eat out and get a healthy meal. Even some rural and inner-city grocery stores have limited fresh and frozen fruits and vegetables. Always politely ask for what you want even though sometimes they might have no idea what you are talking about. Keep asking. You do have a voice and if we all keep demanding chemical-free, whole, plant-based foods, things will slowly change. In some places it's nice to see that they already have changed.

When you have to eat out and the restaurant doesn't have anything on the menu that you will eat, ask for a plate of steamed veggies with nothing on them and a plain baked potato or a salad with a baked potato and a nonfat, vinegar-based dressing. Maybe they have a fresh fruit cup, but sometimes that comes canned in syrup, especially in rural restaurants. If you are going out to a restaurant that you are not sure of, another option is to call ahead before their rush time and see if they are willing to accommodate you. If not, eat before you go. When in doubt about a menu item, always politely ask the server about the ingredients.

Meal Timing

Meal timing is very important to keep you from getting hungry too soon. This along with all the fiber and the nutrient-dense foods that you are eating will keep you from excessively snacking and overeating. The time of day that you eat your meals depends on your schedule. I average five hours between breakfast and lunch, and lunch and dinner.

Breakfast
I like to exercise in the morning before I head to the office (unless I am skiing all day, in which case I eat first). I make sure that I get enough sleep to get up early enough to do this. I have gym equipment in my house for when the weather is bad or I head out for a hike, bike ride, or run when the weather is good. I always drink water first thing in the morning so that I don't become dehydrated. I will also eat a banana or other piece of fruit before I start exercising for instant energy. Within an hour after morning exercising I will fix

myself a big power breakfast such as oatmeal or quinoa with fruit and nuts. Breakfast should contain 400 to 600 calories, which will keep you energized so you will not get hungry until lunch time.

Lunch
Lunch is usually veggies and beans, a large salad with veggies and beans, or leftovers from the night before. Again I try to eat 400 to 600 calories so I am not hungry before dinner time and tempted to snack. If I do get hungry, I snack on fruit.

Dinner
After breakfast and lunch, I have about 800 to 1,200 calories to chow! When you are eating no-oil-added, plant-based food, that's a lot of food! If I need more calories from skiing all day I will add a snack between lunch and dinner, enough to curb my hunger but not too much to sabotage my healthy dinner. This is very satisfying and will keep you energized for the next day!

Spread your meals out as evenly through the day as you can. I know life gets in the way, which is why it is important to be prepared and learn how to pack and carry your meals with you.

I am always amazed when someone tells me that they don't or won't eat breakfast. When you don't eat enough calories for breakfast or lunch, it makes you chase your hunger all day and you will consume way too many calories at night, sometimes without even realizing it. Just because you are eating healthy foods does not mean that you can't overeat if you skip meals, you restrict yourself too much, or your meal timing is off.

Cooking Equipment

I don't recommend nonstick cookware because apparently when heated, the chemicals that the pans are made from get into your food. Cast iron or ceramic are the best way to go. They are inexpensive and seem to last forever.

Learn more about nonstick cookware at willtaft.com (http://willtaft.com/133/health/do-not-use-teflon-cookware)

Here is a list of basic cooking equipment that will help you prepare your meals:
- Microwave oven
- Microwave-safe bowls (non-BPA)

- Assorted sizes of pots and pans
- Electric pressure cooker or crock pot
- Rice cooker
- Bread machine (optional)
- Baking pans for roasting veggies
- Vegetable steamer
- Mandolin
- Food processor
- A good set of knives and a knife sharpener
- Chopping board
- Pot holders
- Measuring cups and spoons
- Mixing bowls
- Colander
- Assorted utensils such as serving spoons, soup ladle, metal spatula, rubber spatulas, can opener, lemon juicer, vegetable peeler, and scissors.

Foods to Have Available

Shopping is fairly simple when you eat healthfully. You don't have to buy exotic foods that you have never heard of, but it is fun to try new food items.

I will list some basic foods that you can have on hand so you always have something healthy to eat.

Fresh and frozen plant-based foods might seem expensive, but when you eliminate so much of the unnecessary stuff that you already eat, you will save a bundle on your grocery bills, not to mention the money you will save on doctors, prescriptions, surgical expenses, and lost time away from work.

Shop by nutrient density, which comes from whole unprocessed fruits, vegetables, legumes, grains, nuts, and seeds. Always read labels, and do not buy anything that has preservatives, artificial flavors, natural flavors (natural flavors are artificial flavors), or trans fats (hydrogenated fats).

This is a starter list of all the food items to have available and a guide for someone who is new to the plant-based eating world. Changing how you cook or learning how to cook is not easy for everyone. It can be fatiguing and frustrating at times. As you practice your cooking using whole, plant-based recipes, you will eventually have your kitchen stocked with only the healthiest foods, and you will be able to make some very tasty and filling meals.

Does natural mean natural? Phil Lempert's article talks about natural flavoring:
http://www.supermarketguru.com/index.cfm/go/sg.viewArticle/articleId/1208

Look for organic fresh and frozen products when possible.

Greens
　　Kale, spinach, Swiss chard, broccoli, Brussels sprouts, dark-leaf lettuce.

Additional vegetables
　　Fresh, local, and seasonal.
　　Frozen, all kinds.
　　Canned low-salt tomatoes (technically a fruit), all varieties.

Fruit
　　Fresh, local, and seasonal.
　　Bananas.
　　Frozen, all kinds with no sugar added.

Legumes
　　Beans, low-salt canned and dried.
　　Lentils and dried peas.

Green and yellow beans.

Grains
Frozen or fresh corn, assorted whole grain flours, quinoa, oatmeal (not quick cooking), whole grain pastas, and brown rice.

Nuts & Seeds (Unsalted)
All kinds (preferably raw), especially English walnuts and ground flax.

Seasonings
All kinds of herbs and spices including Mexican, Italian, and Indian (e.g., curry). Maple syrup and/or agave nectar.

Power Food Recipes

The wonderful thing about cooking with whole foods is that all the recipes can be changed to your tastes or to use up what's in the refrigerator. Be open-minded and experimental. If you are new to cooking or to plant-based cooking, have patience and don't always expect everything to turn out perfect the first time.

*Foods with the asterisk next to them are higher in calories and should be eaten if not to exceed your daily caloric intake. Chocolate pudding is great after a 30-mile bike ride or if you are going cross-country skiing for a few hours. If you don't exercise, don't eat the sweets!

Lunch and Dinner Recipes
Many times my lunch is leftovers from dinner.

Stir Fry Veggies

Chop:
1 pound of mushrooms (Asian mushrooms are good)
2 large carrots
1 celery stalk
1 large onion

6 leaves of Chinese cabbage (Napa)

Sauce:
Mix together:
2 cups of water
2 tablespoons of cornstarch
2 tablespoons of rice vinegar (optional)
2 tablespoons of low-salt soy sauce or Tamari
2 tablespoons of maple syrup
1/2 teaspoon or more of cayenne pepper

Heat your wok or pan until very hot (I use a cast iron pan). Add all the chopped veggies at once. Stir continuously so the veggies don't stick. Cook until they are starting to brown or just becoming tender.
Add 3/4 cup of unsalted peanuts or cashews.
Add the sauce and cook 1 minute or until thickened.
Serve immediately.

Try using a variety of vegetables that you have available! Try it over brown rice.

Tacos

Heat a cast iron skillet until hot.
Place a corn tortilla (with no preservatives) in the skillet and heat for one minute, then flip it over. Carefully layer in the center of the tortilla low-salt nonfat refried beans, hummus, a thin slice of avocado, 1-2 tablespoons of salsa, and 3 organic baby spinach leaves. Continue to heat until the tortilla starts to brown. Remove from the pan, fold in half and let cool for a minute before eating.

To make several, preheat the oven to 200°F and place an ovenproof plate in the oven to warm. Put the folded (or rolled) tacos on the plate to keep warm until you have the desired amount that you want.

Be careful when working around hot pans and plates!

Mushroom Burgers

Put 4 sliced portabella mushrooms, one chopped onion, and one chopped sweet pepper in a large cast iron or ovenproof pan. Roast in a 400° oven for 20 minutes or until mushrooms are cooked.

In a food processor add:
1 can of drained pinto beans (dried with a paper towel)
1 chopped hot pepper
2 peeled garlic cloves
The roasted mushrooms, onions, and pepper
1/2 cup of ground flax seed
Process until blended.

Let this stand in the refrigerator for 1 hour (or longer) to thicken. Heat your frying pan, and add a touch of cooking spray if necessary. Put a large spoonful of mushroom burger in the pan and use the spoon to shape the burger. Cook until browned on both sides.

Serve with tomato slices, spring mix lettuce, homemade hummus, and organic ketchup. Makes 4 large patties.

Kale

1 pound of kale chopped (stems removed)
2 large garlic cloves, minced
1 medium onion, chopped
1 tablespoon of minced fresh ginger
Juice of 1 lime or lemon
Ground black pepper or cayenne

Steam the kale in a vegetable steamer until tender. Sauté garlic, onion, and ginger in a hot pan with a few tablespoons of water until tender. Add kale and stir. Turn off heat and add the lime juice and pepper.

Option: serve with a baked sweet or white potato (skin on).

Soup

Soups and stews are the way to go when you don't have much time. Try to make them the day before you eat them because the flavors of the vegetables and seasonings always taste better after they have had a chance to sit a while.

I rarely put salt in my soups. If it needs salt, I put a little in just before I eat it. My two secret ingredients that I like to use to flavor soups and stews to help avoid using salt are 1-2 tablespoons of maple syrup (per 6 quarts) and chopped hot peppers (to your taste). Other ingredients that I regularly use are onions, garlic, tomatoes, beans, lentils, and assorted veggies. Be creative and keep it simple.

Chili

In a crock pot or pressure cooker:
1 large can of diced tomatoes plus 1 can full of water
1 small can of tomato paste
2 cans of low-salt black or pinto beans with the liquid
1 cup of frozen or fresh corn kernels
1 onion chopped
3 garlic cloves diced
2 tablespoons of maple syrup
1 or more chopped hot peppers
1 seeded and chopped sweet pepper
1 tablespoon of cumin
1 tablespoon of chili powder

1 tablespoon of balsamic vinegar (optional)

Cook on low all day or overnight or according to the crock pot or pressure cooker manufacturer's directions. Serve in a bowl over baby spinach leaves.

Tomato Veggie Soup

1 large or 2 small cans of diced tomatoes
1 can of low-salt chick peas with liquid
1 onion chopped
3 garlic cloves diced
1 large sweet potato chopped
2 medium potatoes chopped
2 teaspoons of oregano
1-2 tablespoons of maple syrup
1 chopped hot pepper or cayenne pepper to taste
Add enough water so everything is just covered.

Cook in crock pot or pressure cooker according to the manufacturer's directions. When the soup is done, add frozen vegetables of your choice such as broccoli or spinach. Cook a few minutes until thawed.

Sweet Potato Stew

1 onion chopped
1 jalapeno pepper diced
1 teaspoon of ground ginger
3 garlic cloves diced
2 teaspoons of ground cumin
1/4 teaspoon of ground cinnamon
1/4 teaspoon of ground coriander
4 medium sweet potatoes peeled and cut into 1-inch chunks
2 cans of chopped tomatoes
2 cans of low-salt pinto or other beans
2 cups of green beans, fresh or frozen
¼ cup of natural peanut butter (optional)

Add enough water as needed to cover your veggies. Put all ingredients into a crock pot or pressure cooker. Follow crock pot or pressure cooker manufacturer's instructions for cooking times.

Roasted Veggies

Preheat oven to 425°.
Spray a baking pan with a thin layer of cooking spray, if needed.

Chop your favorite veggies so they are close to the same size and put in one layer on baking pan.
Roast for 15 minutes. Flip veggies and roast for another 15 minutes or until tender. Veggie suggestions: Potatoes, sweet potatoes, onions, garlic, carrots, Brussels sprouts, cabbage, hot and sweet peppers, mushrooms, and broccoli.

Steamed Veggies

Use the same vegetable size and selection as the roasted veggies (no cooking spray needed). Just put them in a vegetable steamer and follow the steamer manufacturer's directions.

*Pizza**

Dough:
1 1/2 cups of warm water
1 package of yeast
2 1/2 to 3 1/2 cups of whole wheat pastry flour
1 tablespoon of maple syrup
1 teaspoon of salt

Use the dough setting on your bread machine and follow your manufacturer's settings. To make the dough without a bread machine, dissolve yeast in water for 5 minutes. Add the rest of the ingredients with enough flour to make dough easy to knead. Knead on floured counter or board for 10 minutes. Cover dough with a towel and let rise until double.

Punch down dough on a floured surface and shape into the shape of your pizza or baking pan (you can use a floured rolling pin). Cover baking sheet with corn meal or flour before putting the stretched dough on it to keep it from sticking.

Top with 1 small can of tomato sauce mixed with 1-2 teaspoons of maple syrup.
Sprinkle sauce with dried oregano.

Spread 1 box of thawed, drained spinach over the sauce and then top with roasted vegetables such as sweet peppers, onions, garlic, and mushrooms. Evenly dollop tablespoons of your favorite hummus on top of the veggies.

Bake in a preheated 450° oven on the lowest rack for 20-25 minutes or until the crust is well browned.

BBQ Veggies

Barbecue sauce:
2 cups of organic ketchup (Heinz makes one)
1 tablespoon of maple syrup
1/8 to 1/4 cup of white vinegar
Cayenne pepper to taste

Heat these ingredients in a small pot over low heat. Adjust the ingredients to your tastes (I like a lot of vinegar). Serve over roasted or steamed veggies or use as a dipping sauce.

If you like tofu, you can mix some that is extra firm, drained, and cubed into the BBQ sauce. Eat as is or on a whole-grain roll with sautéed (in 2-3 tablespoons of water) peppers and onions.

Mexican Bowl

This is my favorite lunch.
1 handful of organic baby spinach or spring mix salad
1-2 cups of thawed frozen mixed veggies
1/2 cup of low-salt refried or pinto beans
Salsa

Layer in a microwave-safe bowl and microwave until hot (2-3 minutes). You can also add some leftover brown rice or chopped baked potato.

Sushi

The easiest way to learn how to make sushi is to go online to what I call the University of Youtube, (www.youtube.com). Search for "how to make sushi" and you will find many videos to choose from. It takes a little practice but once you get the hang of it, it is quick and easy.

Follow the Youtube recipe using Japanese short-grain brown rice instead of white. Add your favorite raw veggies cut into match sticks (you don't need a lot). Serve with wasabi (it comes in a powder found in the Asian section of your grocery store, just add water) and low-salt soy sauce or Tamari (optional).

Veggie suggestions: Carrots, zucchini, hot peppers, cucumber, avocado, anything leftover.

Green Salad

Start with organic spring mix, romaine, or baby spinach.
Add fresh chopped raw veggies such as sweet peppers, carrots, and cucumbers.
Add a small handful of your favorite unsalted nuts, such as walnuts or almonds.
Add a small handful of your favorite chopped unsalted seeds, such as pumpkin or sunflower seeds.
Add fresh seasonal fruits, such as strawberries, pineapple, or orange segments.
Get creative if you like and top your lettuce with reheated leftovers from last night's dinner.

Top with NNC's salad dressing (page 105) or an all-natural, nonfat salad dressing.

Remember to eat something green and leafy everyday!

Quinoa Salad

This is a great "to go" salad.
Cook 1 cup of quinoa according to package directions (usually a one to two ratio, quinoa to water). Let cool.
Add 1 package of thawed, drained frozen spinach or your favorite greens.
Add an assortment of your favorite veggies, raw, steamed, or roasted.
I like adding roasted sliced mushrooms (raw mushrooms are not digestible), sweet and hot peppers, spinach, onions, and garlic.
Mix in some NNC's salad dressing (see below) to taste. Store leftovers in an airtight container and refrigerate.

NNC's Salad Dressing

1 serving:
Mix together 2-3 tablespoons of balsamic vinegar with a hint of maple syrup. Adjust quantity as needed.

*PBJ!**

2 slices of Ezekiel 4:9 bread (found in the health food freezer section of your grocery store) or a natural 100% whole-grain bread
All-natural peanut butter
No-sugar-added organic jelly or jam (I like Crofter's brand)

Spread the peanut butter on one side of the bread and the jelly on the other. Don't spread too thick because there are a lot of calories in this sandwich. This is great for on the go.

Breakfast Recipes

Oatmeal, Quinoa, or Buckwheat Breakfast

Cook oatmeal, quinoa, or buckwheat on the stovetop or in the microwave according to package directions or to your desired tastes with water or nondairy milk (unflavored almond milk is good).
Add fresh, local, seasonal or frozen fruit, and continue to heat until thawed or warmed.
Add 1 tablespoon of maple syrup, a small handful of walnuts or almonds, and dash of cinnamon (optional).

Toast with Peanut Butter and Jelly

Use all-natural, whole-grain bread toasted with all-natural, low-salt peanut butter and no-sugar-added, organic jelly or jam. Serve with a side of fresh seasonal or thawed frozen fruit.

Sides

Nachos

Spread some organic baked corn chips on a microwave-safe plate.
Top with organic baby spinach leaves.
Top with some leftovers from the Mexican bowl or chili recipes. Or dollop with low-salt, nonfat refried beans.
Dollop evenly with hummus (I like roasted red pepper hummus).
Top with your favorite salsa.
Microwave on high for 1-3 minutes or until warm.
Top with 1/2 an avocado chopped.

Bruschetta

1 whole-grain organic baguette sliced in 1-inch slices
Place baguette slices on a baking sheet and bake in a preheated 350° oven for 15 minutes or until lightly toasted.
Place one small or half of a large basil leaf on each toast slice.
Spread each toast slice with homemade hummus (recipe follows).
Top with seeded chopped tomatoes.

For gluten-free bruschetta, use Mary's Gone Crackers instead of toasted baguettes.

Hummus

You can buy hummus from your grocery store, but make sure you read the ingredients and watch out for too much fat.

In a food processor:

2 cans of low-salt chick peas, reserve the liquid
3 cloves of garlic microwaved until soft, about 15 seconds on high, then removed from the skin
Juice of 1 lemon
1 tablespoon of tahini or peanut butter (optional)

Blend on high, adding reserved bean liquid a little at a time to get a smooth consistency.

Optional: add a chopped roasted red pepper. Use hummus as a vegetable dip or a spread to replace mayonnaise.

Salsa

I like to use store-bought salsa when fresh tomatoes are out of season. Be sure to read the ingredients list first.

Mix together:
1 cup of thawed corn
1 can of black beans, drained and rinsed
1 1/2 cups of diced Roma tomatoes
1/2 cup of diced red onion
1 red bell pepper, seeded and diced
2 teaspoons of minced jalapeno pepper
1 avocado, peeled, pitted, and diced
Juice of 1 or 2 fresh limes (you can also use white vinegar)
1/2 cup of chopped fresh cilantro (optional)
Lightly salt to taste.

Brown Rice

Cook 2 cups of rice (with 4 cups of water) in your rice cooker (or pot with a lid) according to your rice cooker manufacturer's directions.

Options: Add steamed veggies or thawed frozen veggies, 1 or 2 cans of your favorite low-salt beans, and l can of diced tomatoes to your cooked rice for a meal. Serve the plain rice in a bowl with your favorite soup ladled over it. Use the rice in place of the baked corn chips for nachos.

*Fries!**

Don't make too many of these, because they are addictive.
Preheat oven to 425º.
Using 1 potato per person, cut potatoes or sweet potatoes into even slices.
Spread the potatoes in a single layer on a baking sheet (spray lightly with cooking spray if needed).

Bake for 15 minutes, flip fries and bake for 15-20 minutes more or until lightly browned.

Remove from oven and lightly sprinkle with seasoning salt and cayenne pepper (optional).

Microwaved Veggies

Put your favorite frozen veggies in a microwave-safe bowl. Microwave on high, stirring occasionally, until hot.

Sweets and Snacks

Sweet Potato Chips

Use a mandolin or other slicer to slice one peeled small sweet potato very thin. Pat dry with a paper towel. Place in the microwave oven directly on the microwave plate (make sure that it's clean). Microwave on high for 4 minutes, then turn them over. Heat for another 4 to 6 minutes or until brown and crispy.

Try using other vegetables like carrots, beets, white potatoes, or kale. Apples work great too!

Apple Crisp*

Place in a microwave-safe bowl:
1 apple, skin on, cored and sliced thin like for a pie
1 handful of oatmeal
Sprinkle with cinnamon and nutmeg
Add a small handful of walnuts
Drizzle of maple syrup.

Microwave 2-3 minutes until the apples are soft and hot.

Chocolate Pudding*

In a food processor:
Chop 8 oz. of pitted dates for a few minutes.
Add 1/3 of a brick of tofu (about 4 oz.), soft or firm.
Add 2 heaping tablespoons of cocoa powder.

Blend on high until smooth (this may take a while). Add water one tablespoon at a time while blending if it is too dry.

*Snack Mix**

1 cup of Mary's Gone Crackers Chipotle Tomato pretzel sticks, or any spicy, gluten-free pretzels
1/2 cup of unsalted cashews
1/4 cup of shelled unsalted pumpkin seeds
1/2 cup of chopped no-sugar-added dried fruit, like cranberries.

Mix and store in a reclosable plastic bag.

Fruit

Eat a piece of fresh seasonal fruit anytime as a snack!

Hot Fruit

In a microwave-safe bowl:
Add some of your favorite frozen fruit.
Microwave on high until thawed and hot.

For more plant-based recipes:
- International Vegetarian Union's "Recipes Around the World" (www.ivu.org/recipes).
- Fat-free Vegan Recipes (fatfreevegan.com).

Exercise Advice

As you know, exercise is an important part of being healthy. There are many excuses for why people don't do it. Being too busy is a legitimate excuse, but most people who use this excuse are lying (and you know who you are). When you are overweight and you live on junk food, your body is constantly trying to repair itself, which takes a lot of energy. This is the energy that should be used to fuel your day and your workouts. Nutrients are also needed to fuel your body for exercise, but when you don't get enough from living on junk food, finding energy to exercise can be extremely difficult. This is just one of the reasons why people have setbacks, lose their motivation, and quit exercising all together.

What can you do to get motivated to exercise when you just don't like doing it? Start by making dietary changes to whole, plant-based foods. The more junk you eliminate from your diet, the better you will feel and the more motivated you will be to sustain exercise. Pick something that you think you would like to do. Walking is a great start if you live in a climate and a neighborhood that allows it. It is an inexpensive activity, because all you need are some comfortable clothes and a good pair of walking shoes or sneakers. Yoga is another great form of exercise. Taking classes is the best way to go, but if you can't, you can buy DVDs and do it at home. If you own a treadmill or exercise equipment, use it! Start by setting aside a specific amount of time for exercise and slowly increase your time up to one hour per day. When you can exercise for a full hour, start picking up the pace or increase your intensity. Make sure that you exercise with meaning and mindfulness. As you progress, even if very slowly, you will burn calories, develop a healthy body, and be very proud of yourself and who you are becoming.

Another way to stay motivated is to find exercise classes that are available in your area or join a Meetup club (www.meetup.com), like an exercise group or an outdoor adventure club. Changing your routine by the season is a great motivator, because it can keep you from getting burned out and you will look forward to starting the next season's exercise. An example of what I like to do is:

Winter: skiing (alpine, telemark, and cross-country), DVDs for strength training, treadmill, and stair-stepping workouts.

Spring: hiking, running, and cycling (road).
Summer: cycling.
Fall: hiking, running, and strength training.
Year-round: yoga.

    This seasonal training routine really works for my psyche (and the climate that I live in) and it helps me stay motivated year-round. Good coaching is recommended for all sporting activities, even if you are just a recreational athlete.

    How much exercise should you get? A lot has to do with how much time you have for exercising. You should strive for a minimum of one hour of exercise and one hour of being active per day. Some people get confused about the difference between exercising and being active. They are not the same thing. Being active means doing a physical job where you are on your feet a lot, like waiting tables, babysitting young kids, or cleaning your yard. Exercise is where you are stressing your body to push past its previous point of conditioning. If you are extremely overweight, being active is a good start to your exercise program. Start slowly and progress every day.

    Rest and recovery are a very important part of physical conditioning. Many people make the mistake of training without giving their body time to recover from the previous workout. Overtraining can lead to injury and quitting. It is very important to educate yourself about exercise and how to get fit, by working with knowledgeable coaches. Make sure you research the information given to you, because there is just as much bad advice in athletics as there is in dieting.

Do you need to take in extra calories if you are exercising? How many calories you need has many variables to consider, such as age, sex, height, activity, and activity level. There are several online calculators that can help you get a general idea, but they are not always accurate. The Foods to Eat guide staring on page 27 shows that to increase your caloric intake for exercising, it is best done with the increase of grains, starchy vegetables, fruits, nuts, and seeds. Some people tend to overestimate the calories that they are burning during exercise and give themselves permission to eat whatever they want, thinking that they can just burn it off. This usually backfires, results in weight gain, discourages you, and then you quit. Eat good fuel to get maximum results. Seek out plant-based nutritional counseling to get the best results for your caloric intake.

For information on plant-based nutritional counseling, contact Nunda Nutritional Counseling, LLC (www.nundanutrition.com).

The Importance of Nutritional Counseling

Everybody needs help, even when we think that we don't. Seeing your situation through another person's eyes, especially someone who is a professional in their field, can help bring you to some realizations that you might have previously missed.

Look at the big picture. We are not predestined to be sick as we grow old. Today, huge percentages of middle-aged and elderly persons are sick (mainly from poor nutrition and lack of exercise), so we think that it is the luck of the draw whether we get sick or not as we age. It just isn't true. We can age and be healthy at the same time; live a long, happy, productive life; and hopefully die comfortably of natural causes. Whenever I see an active, healthy senior, I am in awe and I hope that I will be so fortunate.

The expense of growing old and being sick is not something we plan for while we are young or at any age. Health insurance is a huge expense in this country, and it does not cover all the medical bills, especially out-of-hospital care and lost time from work, not to mention the financial and emotional burden it puts on your family. Think about it the next time you put a cheap, greasy cheeseburger in your mouth; ask yourself, how much is this really going to cost me?

Getting healthy living and plant-based nutritional counseling can cost a few hundred dollars and save you hundreds of thousands of dollars in future healthcare costs and expenses. Now that's a good investment plan. Try to seek out a good plant-based nutritional counselor or doctor to help you get and stay healthy. Research plant-based nutrition and make getting healthy your new passion. Start a new family tradition. It might just save your life.

For more information contact Nunda Nutritional Counseling, LLC (www.nundanutrition.com).

Summary

Losing weight and living healthfully is a journey. If you are overweight, you are not healthy. There is no way around it. A good way to start getting healthy is to be honest with yourself about your present weight and health situation and then convince yourself that you have what it takes (and you do) and that you are worth it. Treat your health like it is the most precious commodity in the world. Then toughen up and quit with the excuses, because it is change and change is not always easy. You will always run into unforeseen obstacles and setbacks, but this is how we learn, grow, and get results.

Don't expect support, help, or understanding from anyone, especially from people who are closest to you. When you deviate from the norm and take control of your diet and lifestyle, you are threatening those around you just by doing so. When you expect support and don't get it, don't let it take you down, but if you are fortunate and are offered support in your healthy lifestyle endeavors, consider yourself blessed and don't turn it down.

Practice balance in all aspects of your life. Diet and exercise are only a small part of physical and mental health. Discovering your inner drive to take control of your health and discovering what balances your life are what will help you stay on track in your weight-loss journey.

Do you ever think about what your life is going to be like when you are 50, 60, and older? We use aging as an excuse for being fat, sick and being out of shape. We see this as being a part of life because it seems to happen to everyone eventually. It is not necessary to spend our elderly years in bad form, especially now that we have the tools and education to make the best of our lives. It's your choice.

Always remember that when you live healthy and balanced, you will be able to find happiness, fulfillment, and purpose in your life. You will be setting an example and influencing people in a positive manner even if you don't know it. Find strength in your reason for becoming healthy and take pride in doing the right thing.

List of Notable Vegans

This list is from Wikipedia (http://en.wikipedia.org/wiki/Main_Page), of notable vegans from the United States.

André 3000 (rapper)[106]
Carol J. Adams (ecofeminist theorist)[107]
Casey Affleck (actor)[108][109]
Amos Bronson Alcott (teacher, Transcendentalist)[110]
Fiona Apple (singer, songwriter)[111]
Allisyn Ashley Arm (actress, sketch comedienne)[112][113][114]
Emilie Autumn (singer, songwriter, violinist, harpsichordist, poet)[115]
Erykah Badu (singer, songwriter)[116]
Alec Baldwin (actor)[22]
Travis Barker (musician, producer, entrepreneur) [117][118][119]
Neal Barnard (physician)[120]
Gene Baur (activist)[121]
Ed Begley, Jr. (actor)[122]
Brian Bell (guitarist for Weezer)[123]
Steven Best (author)[124]
Mayim Bialik (actress)[125]
Linda Blair (actress)[126]
Peter Bogdanovich (film director)[127]
Sean Brennan (musician)[128][129]
Dan Briggs (musician with Between the Buried and Me)[130]
Patrick O. Brown (biochemist)[131]
Hunter Burgan (Bassist for AFI)[132]
Molly Cameron (Cyclist)[133]
César Chávez (American civil rights activist and co-founder of the National Farm Workers Association)[134][135]
Jessica Chastain (actress) [136]
Robert Cheeke (bodybuilder)[137][138]
Chikezie (*American Idol* finalist and singer)[139]
George Church (scientist)[140]
Greg Cipes (actor, singer, surfer)[141]
Bill Clinton (former president)[142]

Chelsea Clinton (daughter of Bill Clinton)[143]
Kneel Cohn (Singer, guitarist, songwriter for The Dead Stars On Hollywood)[144]
T Cooper (novelist)[145]
Juli Crockett (writer, director, actor, boxer, musician - lead singer of the alt-country band The Evangenitals)[146]
James Cromwell (actor)[147]
Luke Cummo (mixed martial artist)[22]
Bryan Danielson (professional wrestler)[148]
Mac Danzig (professional mixed martial arts fighter)[149][150][151]
Ellen DeGeneres (actress, comedienne, Talk-show host)[10][22]
Thomas Dekker (actor, musician) [152][153][154][155]
Emily Deschanel (actress)[156][157][158]
H. Jay Dinshah (activist)[159]
Michael C. Dorf (Cornell law professor, author)[160]
Michael Dorn (actor)[161]
Lisa Edelstein (actress)[162]
Jade Esteban Estrada (humorist)[163]
William Faith (gothic rock/dark wave artist of Faith and the Muse)[164]
John Feldmann (lead vocalist and guitarist of Goldfinger and producer)[165]
Pamelyn Ferdin (actress)[166]
Adam Fisher (guitarist of Fear Before)[167]
Jon Fitch (professional mixed martial arts fighter)[168][169]
William Clay Ford, Jr. (executive chairman of Ford Motor Company)[22]
Gary Francione (law professor, author)[170]
Michael Franti (Reggae artist)[171]
Kathy Freston (health and wellness author)[172]
Glen E. Friedman (photographer)[173]
Adam Gnade (fiction author)[174]
Brian Greene (scientist)[175]
Michael Greger (physician)[176]
Larry Hagman (actor, producer, director)[177]
John S. Hall (poet, spoken-word artist, lead vocalist of all incarnations of King Missile)[178]
Daryl Hannah (actress)[179]
Bob Harper (personal trainer)[180]
Woody Harrelson (actor)[25][181]
Davey Havok (lead vocalist of AFI and Blaqk Audio)[182]
High Places (Ambient electronic duo, both members)[183]

Jamie Hince (guitarist The Kills)[184]
Chrissie Hynde (singer, songwriter and lead vocalist of The Pretenders)[17][185][186]
Scott Jurek (Runner)[187]
Myq Kaplan (actor, comedian, musician)[188]
Casey Kasem (disc jockey/media personality/voice of Shaggy Rogers)[189][190]
Tonya Kay (dancer)[191][192]
Wade Keller (sports writer - PWTorch / MMATorch founder and editor, radio show host, DVD host)[193]
Anthony Kiedis (singer, songwriter and lead vocalist of Red Hot Chili Peppers)[194]
Jamie Kilstein (comedian/Co-Host of Citizen Radio)[195]
Coretta Scott King (civil rights leader)[196]
Dexter Scott King (activist)[197]
Michael Klaper (physician)[198]
Forrest Kline (lead vocalist of Hellogoodbye)[199][200]
Kathy Kolla (film director)[201]
Dennis Kucinich (Democratic Congressman from Ohio, 2004 & 2008 presidential candidate)[22][202][203]
Carol Leifer (comedienne)[204]
Ted Leo (singer, songwriter and lead vocalist of Ted Leo and the Pharmacists)[205]
Jared Leto (actor)[206]
Carl Lewis (track and field star)[207]
Bob Linden (activist)[208][209]
Howard Lyman[210]
Megan McArdle (journalist and business editor of *The Atlantic*)[211]
Tim McIlrath (singer, songwriter and lead vocalist of Rise Against)[212]
Nellie McKay (actress, animal rights advocate, and musician)[213]
Ian MacKaye (Punk rock singer, songwriter)[214]
John Mackey (CEO)[22]
Tobey Maguire (actor)[215]
Mike Mahler (body-builder)[216][217]
Fred Mascherino (guitarist and vocalist for The Color Fred)[218]
Matisyahu (singer, songwriter)[219]
Josh Max (guitarist and vocalist for The Maxes)[220][221]
Peter Max (artist)[222]
Ed Miller (poker author)[223]

Moby (Electronic musician)[22][105][224]
Isa Chandra Moskowitz (chef and author)[225]
Alison Mosshart (VV in The Kills)[184]
Markos Moulitsas (prominent US political blogger)[226]
Jason Mraz (American singer/songwriter)[227]
Adam Myerson (Cyclist)[228]
Kevin Nealon (actor)[229]
Pat Neshek (Professional Major League Baseball Player)[230]
N.O.R.E. (rapper)[231]
Colleen Patrick-Goudreau (cookbook author and host of the podcast Vegetarian Food for Thought)[232]
Justin Pearson (musician)[233]
Robin Pecknold (lead singer for Fleet Foxes)[234]
Pep Love (rapper in underground hip hop collective, Hieroglyphics) [235]
Joaquin Phoenix (actor)[236][237]
Rain Phoenix (actress)[238]
Summer Phoenix (actress)[241]
Dav Pilkey (children's author)[242]
Dan Piraro (artist)[243]
Brad Pitt (actor, producer)[244]
Prince (singer, songwriter)[245][246]
Princess Superstar (musician)[247][248]
Robin Quivers (Talk-show host)[249]
Randy Randall (guitarist of No Age)[250]
Monica Richards (gothic rock/dark wave artist of Faith and the Muse)[164]
Eric Roberts (actor)[251][252][253][254]
Rikki Rockett (drummer and founding member of Poison)[255]
Omar Rodríguez-López (guitarist for The Mars Volta and At The Drive-In)[256]
Kirsten Rosenberg (singer and writer)[257]
John Salley (professional NBA player)[22][258][259]
Justin Sane (guitarist and vocalist of Anti-Flag)[260]
John Schneider (television actor)[261]
Daniela Sea (actress)[262]
Cindy Sheehan (American anti-war activist)[263]
Jake Shields (professional mixed martial arts fighter)[264]
Alicia Silverstone (actress)[25][265][266]
Russell Simmons (entrepreneur)[22][267]
Grace Slick (Rock musician with The Great Society, Jefferson Airplane, Jefferson Starship, (Starship)[268]

Alex Somers (former member of Parachutes and active member for Jónsi & Alex)[269]
Dean Allen Spunt (vocalist/drummer of No Age)[250]
Jovanka Steele (comedienne, writer)[270]
Steve-O (stunt performer and television personality)[271]
Stic.man (Hip Hop artist with Dead Prez)[272]
Biz Stone (entrepreneur)[22][273]
Salim Stoudamire (Professional NBA Player)[274]
Ruben Studdard (2nd season winner of *American Idol*)[275]
William John Sullivan (software freedom activist, hacker, writer) [276]
Tommy Tallarico (video game music composer)[277]
Ed Templeton (Professional skateboarder)[278][279]
Taryn Terrell (WWE Diva Tiffany)[280][281]
Bob and Jenna Torres (activists)[282]
Will Tuttle (author, speaker, educator, pianist, composer) [283]
Mike Tyson (boxer)[22][284][285]
Jaci Velasquez (Contemporary Christian and pop singer)[286]
Kyle Vincent (singer-songwriter, entertainer)[287][288][289][290]
Alice Walker (Pulitzer prize winning author and feminist)[291]
Billy West (voice actor)[292]
Mike White (scriptwriter)[293]
Persia White (actress)[294]
John Wiese (artist, composer)[295]
Olivia Wilde (actress)[296]
Ricky Williams (American football player)[297][298][299][300]
Saul Williams (Hip hop musician, poet, writer, and actor)[301]
Spice Williams-Crosby (actress and stunt performer)[302]
Venus Williams (Tennis player)[303]
Gretchen Wyler (Broadway actress)[304]
Steve Wynn (entrepreneur)[22]
"Weird Al" Yankovic (singer, songwriter)[305]
Adam Yauch (musician)[306]
David Zabriskie (professional cyclist)[307]
Nick Zinner (guitarist for Yeah Yeah Yeahs)[308]

This is by no means a complete list of notable plant-based/vegans. If you would like to see more names added to this list, please send the information to Wikipedia (http://en.wikipedia.org/wiki/Main_Page).

Resources

Throughout this book you will find several online references to help you continue your education and understanding of healthy, whole, plant-based living. Listed here are also some wonderful resources to help you live your best.

Recommended Websites

For individualized professional nutritional counseling, Nunda Nutritional Counseling, LLC (www.nundanutrition.com).

This website is the gateway to healthy plant based living, vegsource.com (www.vegsource.com).

Dr. Joel Fuhrman, MD, For Superior Health and Your Ideal Weight (www.drfuhrman.com).

Dr. McDougall, MD, Health and Medical Center (www.drmcdougall.com).

John Robbins, Tools, Resources and Inspiration (www.JohnRobbins.info).

Jeff Novick, A Common Sense Approach to Healthful Living (www.Jeffnovick.com).

T. Colin Campbell, Scientific Integrity for Optimal Health (www.tcolincampbell.org).

Rip Esselstyn, 28-Day Save Your Life Plan (www.engine2diet.com).

Chef AJ's Unprocessed, video recipes (www.eatunprocessed.com).

Recommended Books

There are many good whole, plant-based books available. These are some of my favorites:
- *The China Study* by T. Colin Campbell
- *The Food Revolution* by John Robbins
- *No Happy Cows* by John Robbins
- *The Engine 2 Diet* by Rip Esselstyn
- *Prevent and Reverse Heart Disease* by Caldwell B. Esselstyn Jr. MD

- The McDougall Quick and Easy Cookbook, by John A. McDougall, MD and Mary McDougall.

Recommended DVDs

- *Get Healthy Now* and all DVDs by Vegsource.com (www.vegsource.com)
- *Supersize Me,* Morgan Spurlock
- *Processed People,* Mostly Magic Productions
- *Forks Over Knives,* Monica Beach Media.

Made in the USA
Charleston, SC
10 July 2012